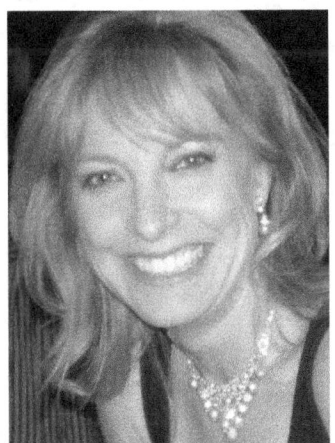

Author: Kathryn Nedved Hoffman

Copyright © 2013 by KAN Publishing, LLC

Published by:

KAN Publishing, LLC

1405 Capitol Dr. Unit C #218

Pewaukee, WI 53072

Website: http://www.Lifewithlymedisease.com

Lyme Disease...
What Your Doctor
Doesn't Know Could Kill You

Table of Contents:

Introduction:

Hello,

My name is Kathryn Nedved Hoffman. Welcome to my world, a world that has been altered by Lyme disease.

The information that I am about to share with you will be life changing. It will either give you peace of mind that you finally realize what is or could be causing your strange symptoms; or you will be completely knowledgeable and understanding of what Lyme disease is, so you can protect yourself and your family from infection.

For those of you who have been told your symptoms are all in your head, you must realize that doctors are human beings and they make mistakes too. Unfortunately, the wrong diagnosis could be fatal. If you have symptoms that doctors can't seem to diagnose, there is hope.

Page 4

General Practitioners don't really understand the many symptoms that come with having Lyme disease. Because of their lack of knowledge, many people spend months and even years searching for a diagnosis. And then you must hope that the diagnosis they give you is accurate.

I was infected while on the job. Like so many, I was one of those people who never got the bull's-eye. But I suspected I had it, because of the many ticks I found on me during the couple of months while we were clearing all the brush, shrubs and debris off a property that my employer was about to build nine homes on.

I went for months without any symptoms at all. I was going mach 10 from the moment my feet hit the floor in the morning, until they lifted back into bed at night. I was active and always very physical in my job and very athletic. I have a girlfriend (Linda) that I went rollerblading with, rock climbing, dancing, you name it. We were both very competitive and so we loved a good physical challenge.

It wasn't until about a year after the bite that I started feeling very fatigued. I remember the back of my neck and shoulders would ache as though I slept wrong. The bottoms of my feet hurt and needed to be rubbed at night so I could go to sleep. Sleep....ah yes, I remember the many sleepless nights too.

They were sleepless, because of the itching on the tops of my feet. The itch was so intense; I finally bought a hair brush to take to bed with me so I could scratch my feet at night. But the more I scratched the more they itched! I had night sweats, and found myself making 4-5 trips to the bathroom every night. That is just not normal…for anyone.

I experienced sudden vision loss and at times even today where my eyes feel like they are connected to a string that is being pulled from side to side. Then there was the *brain fog* as my doctor called it. Like Alzheimer's, I couldn't get the words to come out. I had Days where I couldn't think of the word(s) I wanted to say, or forgetting what I was saying in the middle of a sentence. Then the rashes that would come and go, always showing up in a different place. But it was my eye sight that bothered me the most.

It seemed as though overnight my eyesight just went down the toilet. I had trouble focusing, and I could no longer read up close without having to put on a pair of glasses. I didn't want to admit that my eyes were getting bad, so I went to the Dollar Store and bought 3 different sets of glasses. I bought 1.0, 1.25, and 1.50 prescriptions just to get me through this faze. Prior, my eyesight was always 20/20.

As the Lyme' progressed, the aches and pains would move around the body and become more severe. Some days my lower back would hurt terribly, while other days it was the elbows or hips. But I really knew something was wrong when I woke up one morning and couldn't open my right hand. The thumb muscle was inflamed and my fingers would not move. They were actually curled into an open fist.

That's what prompted me to call my girlfriend Linda. She had just completed a year of Lyme treatment so I thought I would ask her about her symptoms. After speaking with her for just 5 minutes, I knew I had Lyme disease and needed to seek help. Linda had been told by many Doctors that she did not have Lyme disease, as her blood tests all came back negative. She went from doctor to doctor begging for some sort of diagnosis. She even asked one doctor to give her a spinal tap (a very painful procedure) which also came back negative. It wasn't until she was given the name of a specialist did she finally get her answer. It was Lyme disease…exactly what she had suspected. Linda knew the symptoms because her mother had battled Lyme disease for over 35 years. Her mother finally lost her life in December of 2011. She died from congestive heart disease which was accelerated by the Lyme disease. God Bless Lilly.

Knowing what Linda had been through, I decided to see the same specialist. After waiting almost 6 months for an appointment, I was diagnosed immediately based on my symptoms. She also took blood work to verify the Lyme disease, but more importantly, the test results showed I didn't just have Lyme disease….I had many other co-infections that come along with the tick bite that needed to be treated as well.

I too had been tested for Lyme disease 3 times in the past, but my blood work always came back negative. So to finally have a specialist who actually understood Lyme and knew the many symptoms was a miracle in itself.

The doctor told me this was going to be a long recovery and to get my mind wrapped around that idea as quickly as possible. She made it clear that with some of the medication, it would be trial and error to see what would work for me and what would not. But then when I thought the worst of the news was over, she looked at me and explained how this will be in my system for the rest of my life! She said even with antibiotics and other treatment, I will need to be very careful not to over stress my body, or to do too much at one time, or I will start showing these same signs all over again. She even went over a food list of items I could no longer have. *"Lyme disease is a life changer"* she said.

After 14 months of antibiotics and a full regiment of vitamins, herbs, detoxifiers, and drops I finally felt better. I am nowhere near what I consider to be cured, but I have my life back, somewhat. It has been a long road to get where I am today, with a much longer road still ahead of me.

Treatments cost me in access of $32,000.00, and I am not cured. (That was $32,000.00 out of pocket.) What doctors won't tell you, is that Lyme disease is a *"life disease"*, it does stay in your system *forever*, and it is a total *life change* for any person who gets infected. Doctors won't tell you this, because they don't believe it. They believe any person can be cured with just 2-4 weeks of antibiotics. They are *dead wrong,* and for the thousands of patients who have been doctoring for years to get some sort of normality back, the doctors who are not specialists seem to turn and look the other way.

A doctor reading this will deny this completely...unless he or she is a Lyme patient themselves. My doctor has been a Lyme patient since she was a teenager. Because she struggled to find the right treatment for herself, she decided instead of practicing "gut health", she would focus all her attention on curing patients stricken with Lyme disease.

Today her practice is thriving in Morristown, NJ, and people still have to wait months for an appointment to see her. The Northeast and Midwest are *hotbeds* for Lyme disease, but cases have been reported in every state in America. Doctors and scientists are calling this epidemic **worse than the Aids epidemic.**

My story is not over yet. I had to change my life style completely to live with Lyme disease. I struggle every day and hope that my life will someday be normal like it once was. I interviewed over 80 patients before deciding to write this book, and not a single one has been cured, although, many are starting to live with the new form of *normal* while dealing with Lyme disease.

Each case was different, including symptoms, treatments, and time elapsed before diagnosis. But, one thing that we all have in common; we all still have many of the affects from Lyme disease, this is known as *Chronic Lyme.* We have all made life changes in order to cope with the day to day symptoms. If you have been from one doctor to the next with no diagnosis, do not give up! There is hope, and there is help for you.

One thing I must point out to you is that if you have insurance, the insurance companies will only cover the standard 2-4 week antibiotic programs. If you are like me and had the disease for several years before being diagnosed, you had better expect to pay a FORTUNE for medicine and treatment out of pocket.

Understanding insurance companies and what they will cover is like finding a needle in a hay stack at times. But, because Lyme disease is considered an "Infectious disease", many insurance companies will not cover the treatment. Others do not believe that Lyme is serious and therefore, will not cover more than a four week treatment program. So if you are a Chronic Lyme patient...you must expect to pay heavily for treatment. To me, this is one of the biggest insurance scams of the century.

Chapter One:
Lyme disease...perfected and produced by the US Government.

It is true that Lyme disease was produced by our government. This may shock many of you (but then again maybe not), and there will be those who simply will not believe it. You may be asking yourself why would the US government want or need to produce Lyme disease?

The answer is simple...for virological warfare. Yes, I said virological warfare. The disease is reported to have been studied back in the late 1940's. The Nazi scientist who helped to alter this disease completed his research here in America for the US government. After years of research in the US, he then became the head of the research department on Plum Island, just ten miles off the coast of Lyme Connecticut. Hence, the name Lyme disease. Plum Island was a facility that was used by both, the Agriculture department for the study of animal disease research, and the Army as a BW (Bio-Warfare) research facility.

Plum Island was the site used to infect ticks and do bio warfare experiments by Nazi scientists that the US government brought here through a government program called "Project Paperclip". As many as two thousand Nazi scientists were pursued and then contracted by the U.S. government for research and study in the bio-chemical field.

The man accused of being the Lead scientist in charge of Lyme disease is Nazi Erich Traub; a virological and bacteriological expert who worked for the Third Reich's bacterial warfare program during WW II, prior to coming back to the U.S. Traub was lab chief of the Insel Riems which was a secret Nazi biological warfare laboratory. There, he worked directly with Hitler' second man in charge, SS Reischsfuehrer Heinrick Himmler on live germ trials. Near the end of WW ll the US and Soviet Union both raced to hire these German Nazi scientists for post war purposes. Many Nazi scientists brought to the US were granted citizenship in turn for their knowledge and expertise in bio and bacterial chemical warfare.

After the war however, The Soviets ordered Erich Traub to begin research on germ warfare viruses to use on the Russians. Traub became worried for his families safety and planned an elaborate but narrow escape to West Berlin in 1949. Shortly thereafter, Traub and his family came back to the US at which time he continued his research for "Project Paperclip". This information was found in FTR (Failure-To-Report) documents #479 & 480 of government records which were exposed by Disease activist Steven Nostrum and the discovery of Loftus' findings along with his work investigating Plum Island.

Traub was a brilliant scientist who worked under Hitler, and to this day many believe he should have been tried for Nazi war crimes. Traub was a noted authority on viruses and diseases in Germany and Europe, and for that reason he was put in charge of the Third Reich's virological and bacteriological warfare program during World War ll. These Nazi scientists that were brought to the US were supposed to have had only minimal dealings with the Nazi activities, but as information about them unfolded, the findings proved that many of them had very deep dark Nazi party involvement. Our government looked the other way.

Many of the scientists feared retaliation from the Soviets for their Nazi treatment, so they quickly signed contracts with the US government which provided them amnesty in America.

At Plum Island, Erich Traub and other Nazi scientists experimented heavily on the deer tick and the Lone Star Tick which comes from Texas. The tick has a white star on its back giving it the name "Lone Star Tick". Both species are now heavily populated in NY, CT and NJ as well as the upper mid western states such as WI, MN and IL. During Traub' employment, he injected viruses into these ticks in an outdoor lab from 1958-1963 on Plum Island which was visited by as many as 140 species of birds, rodents and white tail deer. Birds often landed at Plum Island to rest during migration in the spring and fall months. The infected ticks were carried off the island by the many species that visited. Heavy winds off shore also carried the diseased ticks to land.

Arial drops of infected ticks were also reported to have been made from planes on several occasions. *The purpose of producing this disease was to slowly infect large populations with assorted symptoms that could be diagnosed as many different illnesses. This was to keep the "virological warfare" from looking like a biologically produced epidemic.* With Lyme disease, each patient is treated differently, and symptoms vary so Doctors become confused and often misdiagnose the real disease. This is truly the perfect "shit storm" for chemical warfare.

Over longer periods of time, the kill rate is high and will decrease the population. For many people with allergies to antibiotics, the fatality rate can be inevitable. Lyme disease is the perfect biological chemical warfare partner for any country looking to expose millions to a fatal disease. Just thousands of infected ticks could act as an incredible army to spread the disease.

Traub had been experimenting with Lyme disease on behalf of the US to use on the Russians during the Cold War. Erich Traub studied at the Rockefeller Institute in Princeton, New Jersey where he perfected his skills with bacteria and viruses before he left the U.S. the night the war began in 1939. While here in the states, Traub was part of the Amerika-Deutscher Volksbund, which was a *"German-American club"*, known to many as *Camp Sigfriend*. The camp ironically was located about thirty miles west of Plum Island in Yaphank, Long Island...which just so happened to be the National Headquarters of the American Nazi movement.

Thanks to our government, Erich Traub got his education right here in the good ole USA before going back to Russia. He excelled in the research there until finally returning to the US where of course the Lyme disease epidemic was birthed. Unfortunately, I don't think they expected it to explode here in the US. *Or, maybe they did?* Perhaps we were meant to be the guinea pigs of their science project, before using it on other countries.

Nazi Erich Traub died in his sleep on May 18, 1985 shortly after having dinner with an old Nazi friend. Are you thinking what I'm thinking here? Either way, I'm glad that man is dead. I don't know how anyone could sleep at night knowing that they perfected an epidemic of mass destruction.

Now keep in mind that Erich Traub did not create Lyme disease. Lyme disease has been around for many years. In fact, a 5300 year old Neolithic frozen mummy that was found in the Alps tested positive for Lyme disease. Erich Traub and other scientists perfected and enhanced the disease and brought it to the level it is today.

Do some research of your own on Scientist Erich Traub. You will quickly find that many other diseases such as "Foot and Mouth" disease and the Aids virus were also developed for chemical warfare, but not necessarily by Traub himself. If this doesn't open your eyes, I would have to say you are living in a comatose state of mind.

Although I could spend my time writing an entire book on Erich Traub and his scientific studies, I choose to spend my time and the rest of this book helping those who have been infected by Lyme disease. I personally hold the US government responsible for the epidemic we are seeing and feeling right here in this country, and globally. Thousands of people are dying each year from this terrible disease. By being misdiagnosed it skews the true numbers of those exposed, which in turn makes Lyme disease seem not to be such a problem to many non-believers...just yet.

Lyme is easily detected in the brain by autopsy, and thousands of people who die each year from what they believed to be something other than Lyme disease could have been saved. Lyme will always show up on an autopsy, but may not be listed as the cause of death on the death certificate. This is why we do not have accurate numbers of those losing their lives each year to a disease that can be *controlled* by simple antibiotics.

It's time people wake up and start looking at the facts...the fact is our Government is responsible for the mass production and release of Lyme disease that has now become the largest epidemic in US history, and soon to be globally.

Page 20

Chapter Two:
Understanding Lyme disease and how you get infected

Lyme disease is a bacterial infection that is transmitted through a tick bite, which to date, is the most common way for a person to be infected. Doctors became familiar with Lyme disease back in 1975, after large groups of children were diagnosed with what doctors called "juvenile rheumatoid arthritis". Ironically, most of the infected children lived in Old Lyme Conn., and a few other neighboring towns.

Through investigations, they realized that a majority of the children lived near heavily wooded areas, which are breeding grounds for ticks. Doctors also noticed that many of the symptoms began to appear in the summer months, which is peak tick season around the country.

Rashes, which are a common symptom, also appeared on the children' bodies before they began to feel arthritic. With further research, investigations showed that blacklegged ticks or (deer ticks) were the cause of this bacterium that is known today as **Borrelia burgdorferi**. This bacterium is spread by the bite of an infected tick. I will discuss this and other bacteria in a later chapter.

Ticks transmit several diseases known as co-infections. The blacklegged tick is most often found on deer, white-footed mice, foxes, squirrels, raccoons, possums, skunks, moles, weasels, chipmunks, birds and horses. These ticks are mostly seen throughout the Northeastern states, and the upper Midwestern states, but have been detected in every state in the country. Ticks such as the brown dog tick, Rocky Mountain wood tick, and American dog tick have not been known to carry the bacterium that causes Lyme disease, but that is now under scrutiny by many in the medical field.

There are four stages of growth for ticks, and at each stage the tick must fill up with blood in order to grow to the next stage in life. The life cycle starts with the eggs. When hatched the tick is in the larva stage, grows to the nymph stage and finally to an adult.

At the nymphet stage the tick is about the size of the period at the end of this sentence. By the 4th stage which is the adult stage, it will be full grown and about the size of a sesame seed. Most tick bites happen during the nymph stage, where the tick is so tiny most folks never see it on them. See photos of ticks and their growth stages near the end of this book.

The tick will attach itself to the human body and usually begins the feeding process after about 24 hours. The tick will feed until the small body becomes engorged and can handle no more. This is the point when the Lyme bacterium is transmitted through the blood stream. If you see a tick that is flat in shape, it has not yet begun the feeding process, and therefore would not have transmitted the bacteria into the bloodstream.

Usually within 7-14 days of the bite, infected persons will notice the *bull's-eye* or red rash on the skin. It is important to know that many people *never* see the bull's-eye or the rash. This is because the rash fades in a short time so many people don't think anything of it, or it is in a place they can't see it, so again, they don't think it's important. If caught early it is easily treated with antibiotics to bring it under control. Left untreated, can be fatal. Treatment varies between patients depending on allergies to medications, how much time elapsed before diagnosis, and the co-infections that the ticks bite carried.

Then, just days or weeks thereafter, you will notice flu like symptoms, fevers, chills, swollen glands, headaches, joint and muscle pain and fatigue. It is important to see a doctor as soon as you can. If possible try to take the tick with you in a jar if you actually find it on your skin.

Time is of the essence when dealing with Lyme disease. If you suspect that you or someone you know may have been infected, early detection can save you from severe health issues associated with Lyme disease and can save you thousands of dollars in medical bills. Most of all...it can save your life. Do NOT under estimate the severity of Lyme disease.

It is also very important that you understand the research and scientific studies that are taking place every day around the globe, to find a cure for this debilitating disease. According to ILADS,

(International Lyme and Associated Disease Society) recent studies show the Lyme disease can be passed along to the fetus during pregnancy which will infect the unborn child. Many children are being born with Autism and doctors around the world are finding the correlations between the two. I'll go further into this later in the book.

Recent studies indicate that Lyme can in fact be sexually transmitted. The carrier may not realize the symptoms, or, may feel they have been cured, but Lyme disease to date has no cure. Therefore, through sexual transmission, individuals who have never shown signs of Lyme disease in the past are now experiencing those debilitating traits. This is a global epidemic.

This causes another problem in and of itself. Those being infected by their sexual partners may experience symptoms but those symptoms may not be nearly as severe as those felt and experienced by the carrier who passed the disease along. Can you just imagine if you have a sexually active carrier who doesn't know he/she has Lyme, out in the public sleeping with every

Jane, Beth and Mary or every Tom, Dick or Harry they meet?

For many infected through sexual transmission, they may never make the correlation between the two, so more than likely they will never suspect they have Lyme disease and therefore will never ask their doctor to test for it. This could go on for generations. Many will be diagnosed through the correct blood tests while tens of thousands and even millions of people will go undetected, untested, and untreated. Lyme disease can and probably will be the epidemic that wipes out millions of our population.

Another issue that arises is the meat that we purchase in the grocery stores and super markets. Just think for a moment, if a deer, cow, sheep, pig etc. gets infected by a tick bite, wouldn't that meat be contaminated? The answer is yes. Unless you cook the meat completely well done where the bacteria has been killed off, if anyone eats a piece of meat that is rare, medium rare or even medium, they are ingesting meat that is still blood red and has not killed off the Lyme bacterium. Now we have a serious problem. I have asked this question to several Lyme specialists and none of them really know how to answer it. However, once I pose the question to them, you can physically see their facial expressions change, almost as if they have never thought about that possibility.

As a person who has been living with this debilitating disease, I think of everything. Now, if we know that you can get infected through your sexual partner, and that unborn children can be infected through the fetus, why couldn't we be infected through the meat that we eat if it is still rare or bloody?

Many people will be infected because of blood transfusions. Even those folks who donate blood and feel they are doing something wonderful could in fact be infecting others. Testing for the Lyme co-infections is the key to detecting this disease.

I'm sure there may be other ways that we can get infected by this terrible disease, but we just haven't realized them yet. This is an ongoing epidemic, and one that is impossible to stop unless every person was to receive some sort of vaccination. But again, as of today, there is no vaccine available to cure Lyme disease.

Chapter Three:
How to protect yourself from getting Lyme disease

It is always best to be proactive when dealing with any disease, however since Lyme disease has become such an epidemic, constant care must be taken to avoid tick bites.

The best way to protect yourself and your family is to always wear light colored clothing when working or enjoying the great outdoors. Be sure to wear enclosed shoes and socks that you can tuck the bottom of your pants into. It is best to wear long sleeves and tuck the shirt into your pants. In the heat of summer, a long sleeve cotton shirt is breathable and very comfortable and can protect your arms. Hats are also good as it takes quite a bit of time to find ticks in the hair. On the scalp it's like trying to find a needle in a hay stack.

Now, if you're like me you have no desire to dress in long sleeves or pants that you will tuck into socks in the summer. Especially on those hot and humid days…wearing clothes at all is a drag! You constantly have to take showers or stay in air conditioned rooms so you don't sweat. So if you wear shorts and sandals, be sure to protect the skin.

If you have any unprotected skin areas, such as legs, arms and feet due to wearing shorts or sandals, be sure to use a repellant that contains DEET. This is especially important on those hot summer days when you are in and out. All exposed skin should be sprayed or rubbed with some sort of repellent.

It is also important to remember to walk in the center of paths or on sidewalks rather than the grassy areas. Ticks will find their way to leafy areas, or areas where there may be dead grass or clippings after mowing the lawn. So once you have completed your weekly yard maintenance, be sure to rake and bag all debris. Do not leave piles of branches, leaves, grass or weeds in or around your yard, as this will quickly become a great nesting place for the ticks. Once you have the debris in a bag, tie it tightly and place it into the trash can for pick up.

If you love to garden like I do, make certain you take your shoes off outside or wipe them down with a white cloth before taking them inside your home. You should always remove the clothes you were wearing and check them for ticks before throwing them into the wash machine. Also check all exposed skin areas and if need be, have a loved one spend a few minutes checking your scalp and body for any signs of the little critters.

If you have a patio or deck near any trees, you want to keep it as clean as possible to keep ticks at bay. A weekly wash down with your garden hose will keep the ticks off patio furniture and the surrounding area. For those of you who love to have bird feeders in your yard…..you many want to think twice. Seeds that fall to the ground make a great feeding place for squirrels, rodents and many other animals. Ticks thrive in this type of environment, and use those areas to find the next "host" for them to both feed and travel on.

Those animals can also carry ticks into your yard, and that is what you want to avoid most. Remember, in order to help avoid infection you must be proactive.

It's like having a bus pull up to your front door and dropping off an epidemic. Those bird feeders are like bus stops! Always be mindful of not running in and out of the house for phone calls, to get drinks or forgotten items without taking off your shoes first.

For those of you women who decide to have children, before getting pregnant, have a blood test taken to be sure your blood is free and clear of the infection. If you find you have Lyme in your blood, speak to a specialist before getting pregnant, especially since Lyme and childhood autism are being linked together. Do your homework and research and read all that you can before making that important decision to bring a child into this world. It would be devastating to give your unborn child a death sentence when it could be prevented. I also cannot imagine anyone wanting to give birth to an Autistic child if they can prevent it. Hell, it's hard enough to raise healthy kids, much less a child born with a disease of any kind.

As for sexual transmission of Lyme disease, act responsible. If you know you have Lyme disease, it is up to you to take precaution with your sexual partner(s) and be open about the information. It is also very important that you discuss this with a specialist and not just your family doctor or Gynecologist. Too many doctors dismiss this information as crap, rather than spending some serious time doing their own research and speaking with Lyme specialists around the globe. Lyme disease is an epidemic and must be treated as one.

You must also be diligent about keeping a close eye on your pets so they don't carry ticks in to the house. I take two minutes to wipe my dogs down every time they go out in the yard and come back inside. Just using a damp cloth to rub across their entire body and under cage as well as their legs and paws will take off any pollen and also help me to see if they are clean of ticks or other insects. This is a good practice for dogs and cats.

Don't forget to keep your pets up to date with a good tick and flea collar, or by using products like *"Frontline"* which is what I use on my dogs to help protect them all year round. Protecting your pets is as important as protecting yourself.

If you do think you may have been infected call your doctor immediately and have them take a blood test to verify. If you have the rash or bull's-eye, that is even better for the doctor to diagnose. But it is imperative that the Doctor get you on antibiotics *immediately.*

There are several ways that ticks can get onto your body or your dogs. Obviously, they will attach themselves to your clothing or skin if you happen to walk on the grass or in grassy areas. Leaning up against a tree or sitting under one, as they can drop onto your body. The wind can blow them a very long distance.

When I visit one of my girlfriends, she happens to live in a house surrounded by wooded areas. Every time I have been there, if we sit at the pool or on her patio, the wind carries the ticks from the trees and woods and I always find at least one on me when I leave.

My friend also has a large fence of cut wood for their fireplace. Wood piles are such breeding grounds for ticks, and they can literally be carried right into the house on the wood. If they drop on the floor while bringing the wood in, you just caused yourself a disaster.

Even her dog has to be checked for ticks daily, as just letting the dog out to go to the bathroom, or to run around the yard, he/she can pick up several and come bouncing with them on the fur back into the home. So no matter where you live, always be aware that they could be present.

Chapter Four:
Why doctors misdiagnose Lyme disease

Lyme disease has been called *"the great imitator"* because it imitates so many other diseases, leaving doctors convinced that you may have for example: MS (Muscular Dystrophy), instead of Lyme disease. This misdiagnosis happens more often than people realize. We will talk more about the other misdiagnoses in another chapter.

Lyme disease and the co-infections move around the body relatively quickly, and affect different areas of the body. Because each case is different and affects patients differently, doctors have a very difficult time diagnosing Lyme, therefore causing misdiagnosis. Treating a misdiagnosed disease could be fatal.

So patients ask "Why don't doctors just take blood tests to get the correct diagnosis"? Well if it was that simple, there would not be any misdiagnosed patients. Fifty-seven patients I interviewed were told their blood work tested negative for Lyme disease. All of them had taken between 2-5 blood tests. The problem here is that there are too many false-negatives with the blood tests.

False-negatives are false readings showing a negative reply to the disease. I was tested three times and all three blood tests came back negative. I thought how could this be? According to several specialists, Lyme disease can creep into the bloodstream and lay dormant for weeks, months and even years. You can live with it comfortably and never know you have it, until one day you do something that wakes up this sleeping giant. Once you wake it up or piss it off, the "life change" begins. Game on!

The *Borrelia burgdorferi* bacterium looks like a cork screw. It literally attacks the blood cells and burrows itself into the cell where it will either lay dormant or will continue to go from one cell to the next infecting each cell as it travels. The reason it is so hard to treat is because our blood cells have a protective layer surrounding it. Once the bacterium breaks through that protective layer, the cell immediately protects it, thinking it is part of the cell.

This means for many, that being on antibiotics could take up to 18 months of treatment to hit the bacterium hard. If it stays inside the cell dormant, it is protected and never gets treated by the medicine. It has to be on the move to get attacked itself. If it moves from one cell to the next, it gets hit with the medication each time it leaves the cell. It can take a long time to get the bacterium under control at that rate.

Doctors however, know that long term treatment with antibiotics can cause many other harmful issues. Kidney and liver damage as well as Gall bladder problems, just to name a few. Also, it is possible to become immune to the medicine where the body will no longer react. This is why doctors find themselves switching up the medications and thru trial and error hopefully get it under control.

My girlfriend Linda is living proof that Lyme disease can lay dormant in the body. She had three blood tests and a spinal tap and all came back negative. She had the Lyme virus in her bloodstream for 7-10 years before she was ever diagnosed with the disease. She was always very athletic so her body was always getting large doses of oxygen....the one thing that Lyme disease *doesn't like*. A well oxygenated body can keep the monster dormant for a very long time. Exercise is crucial.

In Linda's case, her work schedule had become very busy so she wasn't getting the same amount of exercise that she once did, leaving the body less oxygenated. So of course less oxygen woke up the virus and then the "life change" began.

Linda had a very bad case of Lyme. For her, treatment consisted of antibiotics, fed thru an IV Pick or through intravenous that went from her arm directly into her heart for an entire year. She also had daily doses of herbs, vitamins, drops and homeopathic concoctions she would make at home. She also had her Appendix removed shortly after her treatment stopped.

Now in Linda's case, her kidney, liver and gallbladder were all being protected by the different medications. However, all the toxins and antibiotics then over flowed into her appendix because they had no other place to go. This caused her appendix to fail, which resulted in her having it removed.

It's been over two years since her treatment, and every day is a struggle in some form, but she is leading as normal of a life as she can. Lyme disease is a total life change if you are one who has had it in your bloodstream for months and even years. Before Linda even realized she had the disease, she got pregnant and her boys are now showing signs as well.

Lyme disease would be easy to diagnose if all patients had the same symptoms. Now that would just be too easy. The problem people have is that the symptoms vary from patient to patient. Some come and go so quickly, many don't even realize it's a symptom. Rashes for example; will come and go sometimes within a few days. Aches and pains will affect one body part one day and another body part the next, and then disappears for months before returning. This is what causes so much confusion and misdiagnosis by doctors.

I will constantly repeat myself and tell everyone; timing is crucial when you have been infected. As soon as you see the bull's-eye or the rash, or start feeling weird or strange symptoms, get yourself to a doctor. If your blood work shows negative, get a second opinion. It is best to seek out a specialist who only deals with Lyme disease. They are more aware of the many symptoms and strange patterns that occur.

The best way to track your symptoms is simply to keep a log. You need to write down anything on your body that hurts, itches, feels weird and even seems stupid. Doctors (specialists) need to know these things in order to diagnose this disease properly.

Although there are many labs in the country that will test for Lyme disease, there is only a few that specialize in Lyme testing. My Specialist sent my blood work to a lab in Chicago for the initial diagnosis. The ELSA test is only 65% accurate in the detection of Lyme disease. That means 35% of patients get false-negative readings. This is not good. A test should be at least 95% sensitive to pick up a reading. This is just another reason why testing for co-infections is so important. To date, there are 11 different species of ticks found carrying the bacterium. However, the current test only works with one species. If your test for Lyme comes back negative, but your Q-fever or Babesia testing comes back positive, it's a sure thing your doctor is going to see that you have Lyme. Scientist Erich Traub dam sure knew what he was doing when he perfected this disease! It truly presents a cluster f_ck for doctors to pin point and treat.

Most doctors, unless they are Lyme specialists, only check for Lyme disease and never bother to check for the co-infections. For this reason alone, so many people are misdiagnosed. In my case, the reason my blood tests came back negative was because the doctors never had the blood tested for *Babesiosis (Babesia); Bartonella; tick-borne relapsing fever Borrelia; Brucella; Colorado tick fever virus; Ehrlichia; Mycoplasmas; Powassan encephalitis virus; Q-Fever; Rocky Mountain spotted fever (Rickettsia); Tularemia (bacteria).*

Unfortunately, I had three co-infections which would have alerted a specialist that I had Lyme disease. However, specialists do know that they still have not uncovered all the co infections that come with Lyme. Tick-borne infections weaken the immune system which allows opportunity for other infections to wreak havoc on your system. This makes it difficult to diagnose the disease and can also result in a very long recovery time. One more piece to this agonizing puzzle. Ugh.

In addition to these co infections there are diseases that are widespread in the environment, such as CMV (Cytomegalovirus), EBV (Epstein Barr Virus) and HHV-6 (Human Herpes Virus). Although these diseases may not necessarily be contracted from tick bites, a specialist may need to run PCR tests (Polymerase Chain Reaction) on these rather than the usual antibody tests for the co-infections. Many people also have infections from high levels of toxic metals. I had very high levels of lead in my bloodstream which my doctor had to treat as well. I was amazed at the symptoms I had just from the lead!

I had to detoxify my body of lead while taking all the other medicines. At one point I was taking 23 different herbs, vitamins, drops and antibiotics at one time. Talk about confusing! Can you just imagine how difficult it was to keep track of all this medicine when I was dealing with brain fog? Some had to be refrigerated, others not. Some had to be taken 2-3 times a day, and others only once a week. I felt like I was being pickled! My body was so out of sorts, I didn't know from day to day if I was going to have a normal bowl movement or if I was going to have 5 that day. It was a real special time for me. And to top it all off, my friend Hala called me a Sphincter! Yeah…it made me laugh, but not feel better.

One thing is certain, be sure you seek help from a specialist if your doctor is coming up with negative results. I believe it is always good to get a second opinion. And of course, don't be afraid to ask your doctor to check the blood for co-infections. It is also essential to have your doctor check for Zinc, vitamin B and vitamin D levels. These are so important to help with your recovery. Most patients are lacking in these vitamin and minerals which will prolong the treatment if they are low. My vitamin D level was extremely low, and I felt better after one week of being on it.

Many doctors are not even aware of the co-infections that come along with the Lyme disease. If your doctor asks you what co-infections you want to be tested for….get up and leave. Or, if he/she says they don't know of any so called co-infections, again, get up and leave. And finally, if your doctor sees the bulls-eye and still tells you after the blood test that you don't have Lyme disease, that it is all in your head....oh PLEASE walk out. That is not the right doctor for you. Any time you go into a Doctor' office with the tick bite/bulls-eye and or the actual tick, your doctor should immediately give you a prescription for antibiotics.

I've actually seen patients who went to the doctor with a full blown bulls-eye on their arm or leg, and in one case the patient presented the tick she removed from the leg bite. Her doctor told her not to worry and to watch it for a few days. If the bulls-eye went away, she would be fine! Are you kidding me?!?!? That doctor should have been SHOT! Antibiotics MUST start immediately. Period. Don't let a doctor inflict a death sentence upon you because he/she is misinformed, or doesn't believe that Lyme disease is actually a *real and serious disease.*

Treatment can be tricky, as antibiotics may help to control or cure one co-infection, but may not work on others. Each co-infection requires its own treatment.

Only a Lyme specialist can truly work with you to find the best treatment for your case.

This too is why doctors have trouble diagnosing Lyme disease. Even if your blood test results are positive for Lyme, the antibiotic you are given may not be the correct antibiotic to cure your specific symptoms. It is crucial for your doctor to know which if any co-infections you have, and what medicine you need to get started on. Don't be surprised if the doctor has you switching medications throughout the course of your treatment; this is normal. The doctor may have to raise or lower certain medicines in order to fight off the different infections. And if you have allergies to any of the antibiotics, you may have to heal yourself through a series of holistic treatments and no antibiotics at all.

To truly help your doctor make the correct diagnosis, you will be asked many questions about your symptoms. It is imperative that you be as specific as you can in telling your doctor what has been going on differently in your body. So if you suspect you may have Lyme disease, write down all the different aches and pains you have noticed, or any other crazy symptom that you have not previously experienced. Even if you think the doctor is going to tell you you're nuts.....say it like it is. Your notes and log book could save your life.

In fact, I'll go one further…get a log book and for 30 days write down in that book (religiously every day) what your body is feeling. If you have no aches, pains or anything write it down. If you have a slight headache for just 15 minutes, write it down. Be specific with your ailments and try to write clearly about each symptom so the doctor will understand what you felt and where the problem was. (i.e., arm, leg, back, lower back, shoulders, etc.)

When I went to see my specialist for the first time, she asked me what my symptoms were. The first thing I told her was; "Doc, you're going to think I'm crazy for saying this, but…." She laughed and replied, "I know you must have Lyme disease, every patient that comes here says the same thing to me…I'm used to hearing it." Then she proceeded to type my symptoms into her laptop, and she asked me if I had felt this or that….and some I had totally forgotten about until she brought them up.

I thought I was nuts telling my doctor that the top of my feet itched so badly I had a hard time sleeping. Or the fact that I was getting up to go the bathroom 3 and 4 times a night. Who would have ever known these were symptoms of Lyme disease, unless you've experienced it firsthand? God Bless my doctor! I would have never thought to even bring those things to her attention. It never occurred to me that getting up to go to the bathroom 2-3-4 times a night was a problem. I just assumed I was drinking too many liquids before going to bed. When my girlfriend Linda experienced that, she was pregnant and thought it was normal during pregnancy.

At the end of the day, you know your body better than anyone else….including your doctor. What you tell your doctor will determine what medication if any he/she needs to put you on. So get your pen and paper ready and make notes of all your weird symptoms…no matter how crazy you think it sounds. And I am serious! Even if your crap is neon pink that day, write it down. If you have a hard little bump under the skin on your chin and it itches, mention it. Don't leave anything out or you could be misdiagnosed.

Chapter 5:
The most common recorded symptoms of Lyme disease

There are many recorded symptoms of Lyme disease, and I will discuss those with you in this chapter. Keep in mind however that each year that goes by, results in new symptoms showing up. The environment is always changing and new forms of bacteria are being discovered.

As discussed earlier, the most common symptoms are the bull's-eye and the rash. Not all people get the bull's-eye or see the rash. I had no sign of either when I got the bite, and working outside like I did, I was diligent in always checking my body for ticks each day after work. The rash for me came much later in time. When it did show up, it appeared on my chest for a week then disappeared. Then, a few weeks later is showed up on my waistline. The rash would come and go but always in a different location and for a different amount of time.

Headaches, joint and muscle pain and chills are all very common. Some patients have severe migraine type headaches while others do not. Headaches are quite common among Lyme patients. Joint and muscle pain range depending on the person, but many complained of knee, neck, shoulder and lower back pain. For me personally, the neck, shoulder and lower back were always in pain. Common Inflammation of the thumb muscle tissue, knees, elbows and wrists occurred. Flu Like symptoms occur in many cases.

Foot pain is a common symptom. The bottoms of the feet will hurt, making walking a miserable task, while the top of the feet (instep) area will itch terribly. General body itch is also common. The back, legs, arms itch uncontrollably.

Night sweats, low grade fevers (hot flashes) and sleep disturbance became common place. Waking up several times throughout the night to go to the bathroom, more than once is not normal unless pregnant. Swollen glands, sore throat, ear aches, lightheadedness, dizziness, fatigue, abdominal pain, chest pain and heart palpitations.

Many patients experienced diarrhea, memory loss and poor concentration, myalgia, irritability, mood swings and depression, Tinnitus, vertigo, testicular/pelvic pain, facial numbness or pain, cranial nerve disturbance or neurological ticks, palsy and optic issues. *And people wonder why doctors have a difficult time diagnosing Lyme disease!*

One of the most common symptoms experienced was fatigue. I personally could not walk up *two steps* without sitting down to catch a breath. I had days where it would take me a half hour to walk up the thirteen steps to get to my bedroom just to lay down. I would go to sleep at 7pm exhausted, and wake up feeling the same way after sleeping for twelve hours! I had no energy and if I tried to do something physical, it would not take longer than a few seconds before I had to stop. For someone who is normally very active and physical…this was devastating.

I, like so many other patients experienced neurological twitches and ticks that I never had before. The symptoms are so vast that it is a wonder at all that patients are being diagnosed correctly.

Lesions on the brain are also very common with Lyme disease. Unfortunately, many people don't

---

know they have them until an MRI is taken or an autopsy after death. Many people who have passed from a diagnosis other than Lyme disease, have shown to have lesions on the brain, which lead to the conclusion that the individual had Lyme disease present in their system at the time of death.

The one thing I do know for certain is this; if you see a specialist instead of a family practitioner, through questioning and a thorough examination, commonalities with your symptoms will prompt the specialist to take blood and send it to the lab.

The specialists that I spoke to sent the blood work to one of two laboratories in the country; either Chicago or Arizona where labs specialize in Lyme screening. This is pertinent for a proper diagnosis. It is for this reason that I highly recommend a specialist. Now don't get me wrong, some family practitioners and pediatric doctors can do the test as well, however, the lab it is sent to is as critical as making the diagnosis.

And again, unless the doctor/specialist is checking for some of the normally associated co-infections, you could end up with a false-negative reading. Before I go into the co-infections of Lyme disease it's really important for you to see what other diseases people are being *misdiagnosed* with having. The following pages will give you a glimpse at why Lyme disease is so hard to diagnose. Take special note of the symptoms of each of these diseases and then look at the Lyme symptoms.

Chapter Six:
The most common misdiagnosis of Lyme disease

First, nobody wants to hear that they have a *disease*. Disease is like a dirty word, and people have a hard time adjusting to the fact that they could have a disease. It's equivalent to walking around with really bad body odor. Who wants that?! And more importantly, who wants to even get close to you or hold your hand or sit next to you? However, I am going to walk you through the many diseases that patients around the country have been misdiagnosed with. As you read about each disease, you will see how many symptoms are *like* those associated with Lyme disease. Remember Lyme disease is considered *"the great imitator"*.

One of the most commonly misdiagnosed diseases is *MS (Muscular Dystrophy)*. MS is an inflammatory disease. The myelin sheaths surround the brain and spinal cord becomes damaged, which leads to the loss of myelin and scarring. The cause is either the failure of myelin producing cells or the destruction of the immune system. *Symptoms associated with MS that are also seen in Lyme disease are:*

- Fatigue
- Weakness
- Numbness
- Muscle spasms
- Constipation
- Frequent need to urinate
- Double vision
- Eye discomfort
- Vision loss
- Uncontrollable rapid eye movements
- Facial pain
- Depression
- Dizziness
- Hearing loss

Fibromyalgia: Other than osteoarthritis, Fibromyalgia is the most common musculoskeletal condition. It is still very often misdiagnosed and still very misunderstood. It is most commonly known for its terrible fatigue and widespread muscle and joint pain. Other symptoms of Fibromyalgia that are similar to Lyme disease are:

- Chronic muscle pain
- Muscle spasms or tightness.
- Moderate to severe fatigue
- Decreased energy
- Insomnia
- Waking up as tired as when you went to sleep
- Body stiffness
- Brain fog
- Abdominal pain
- Nausea, bloating
- Constipation or diarrhea (Irritable bowel syndrome)
- Tension or migraine headaches
- Facial and/or Jaw tenderness
- Sensitivity to light, cold, noise, medicine or odors
- Depression
- Tingling or numbness in the hands, arms legs, feet or face
- Increased urinary frequency

Page 56

- Feeling of swelling in the hands and feet

Alzheimer's disease: It is a type of dementia that causes problems with memory, thinking and behavior. The symptoms usually develop slowly and get worse over time, which interfere with day to day activities. Alzheimer's disease is not part of getting older as many people say it is. Symptoms of Alzheimer's disease are:

- Memory loss or brain fog
- Difficulty with concentration
- Confusion
- Vision problems
- Loss of words during conversation
- Mood swings
- Change in personality

Chronic Fatigue Syndrome: This is a complicated disease and the cause is unknown. Extreme fatigue ***may*** be caused by mental or physical activities, and rest will not make it better. Some theories are that it could be caused by anything from a viral infection to psychological stress. There is no single test to diagnose Chronic Fatigue Syndrome. The following symptoms associated with Chronic Fatigue Syndrome are also similar to Lyme disease.

- Low grade fever
- Vision loss, blurring, eye pain & dry eyes
- Chills & night sweats or excessive sweating
- Rashes
- Dry mouth & eyes
- Ringing in the ears, Tinnitus
- Unexplained weight changes
- Twitching of the muscles
- Recurring Infections

Lupus: No two cases of Lupus are the same. Symptoms can come and go quickly or be brought on slowly. They can be temporary or permanent. Cases can be either mild or severe, and generally people will get flare-ups, and sometimes get worse than others, and even disappear for a short time or for a very long period of time before returning. This sounds so crazy, I'm wondering how the hell doctors even came up with this! In my mind you either have it or you don't.

Sounds like the Hokey Pokey...it's my arm... no it's my leg...no it's neither.

Symptoms of Lupus that are also similar to Lyme disease are:

- Fatigue and fever
- Joint pain, stiffness and/or swelling
- Headaches, confusion and memory loss
- Skin lesions that seem to worsen with exposure to sun
- Shortness of breath
- Butterfly-Shaped rash on the face that will cover the cheeks and bridge of the nose
- Chest pain
- Dry Eyes
- Fingers and toes turn white or blue when exposed to the cold

Rheumatoid Arthritis: In the early stages, it will affect the smaller joints first, such as those that connect the fingers to the hands and the toes to the feet. As the arthritis progresses through the body, it will then affect the ankles, knees, hips, shoulders and elbows. Usually these symptoms will occur in the same joints on both sides of your body. Rheumatoid arthritis symptoms will come and go and the severity may increase or decrease. People experience "flares", or "flare ups" but then will many times experience remission. Over time, it can cause the joints to shift out of place and even deformity. Symptoms of Rheumatoid Arthritis that are also similar to Lyme disease are:

- Tender, stiff, warm or swollen joints.
- Fatigue
- Muscle aches
- Loss of appetite and weight loss
- Firm bumps of tissue under the skin of the arms (rheumatoid nodules)
- Fevers

Celiac Disease: This disease has about 300 different symptoms and affects each person differently. The symptoms are so vast, that it often gets confused for *irritable bowel syndrome* or *lactose intolerance.* Some of the symptoms associated with Celiac disease that are also similar to Lyme disease are:

- Fatigue
- Abdominal bloating and pain
- Diarrhea
- Irritability
- Chronic constipation
- Weight loss
- Joint pain

Addison Disease: Is caused by a hormonal disorder that can affect both male and females of all age groups. Addison disease occurs when the adrenal glands don't produce enough of the hormone called "Cortisol" and sometimes the hormone called "Aldosterone". Symptoms of Addison disease that are also similar to Lyme disease are:

- Severe fatigue
- Muscle weakness and pain
- Joint pain
- Nausea
- Weight loss
- Lower back pain
- Diarrhea

Other diseases that are also very similar to Lyme disease symptoms can be found in PD (Parkinson's disease), pulmonary embolism, Syphilis, Nocardiosis, Tuberculosis, Irritable bowel syndrome, and Anxiety.

This list is only a handful of the different diseases that are similar to Lyme disease. If you look at each of them carefully, you will notice several of the same symptoms that show up in each disease. Keep in mind that I did not list *every* symptom for each disease, because the lists seem to go on forever.

I'm sure by now you are starting to understand why so many people are misdiagnosed every day. I believe that the majority being misdiagnosed are being told they either have MS, Fibromyalgia and Alzheimer's. These three diseases are almost identical to Lyme disease under a microscope. It takes a really thorough analyst to spot the difference between the four. If you do a little homework, you will find that in the last 10 years, the number of MS and Fibromyalgia cases have radically increased. Knowing what I know about Lyme disease, I would bet that the majority of those people have been misdiagnosed. And, if those people had blood tests taken today for "co-infections" of Lyme disease, those current statistics for MS and Fibromyalgia would drop tremendously, while the numbers of Lyme patients would shoot through the roof.

And once again I will repeat myself…get a second or even third opinion. Do not accept a doctor's diagnosis until you have had blood work tested for *Lyme co-infections*.

Chapter 7
You've been diagnosed with Lyme; now what happens:

So you're one of the lucky who found a specialist who tested the blood for co-infections. And you test positive. Now what? Well, wipe that dumbfounded look off your face and take a deep breath. You need to come to the realization right here and right now that this is a lifetime disease....so buck up buttercup and settle in for a long haul.

Getting well is not going to be easy, and there may be days (many days) where you feel like dying. But you're going to get your sorry butt up and do what you can to have even a little bit of normality until the medicine takes hold of the bacteria in your body, and you begin to feel better. Understand this; if you've had Lyme disease for some time (several months or even years) you can expect that it will take 1-2 years to feel better and maybe even longer than that. Yes...it can take that long, and I refuse to sugarcoat anything about this dam disease.

This is why you must mentally prepare yourself the moment you get the shit news handed to you from your doctor. It's not the end of the world unless you want it to be. For me, I suspected I had it, so when my doctor confirmed it with me I was relieved to know I finally had a diagnosis for everything weird that was going on with my body.

Once your doctor has given you the wonderful news, he/she will discuss treatment(s) with you depending on your specific situation. Each case is different. Just because Mary or Bob down the street or a coworker has it doesn't mean you should ask them what they did or what medicine they took. You are unique and will need to help the doctor determine what works best for you.

Your constant participation with the doctor will make all the difference in the world. This is the time when you need to really keep good notes about your body and how you feel from day to day. That is the only way to know if the medicine you are prescribed is actually working. Now most patients start out with a prescription of Doxycycline, but...if you have allergies to medicines, you may be given something else.

I personally was on doxycycline for 14 months. The doctor also gave me prescriptions for Cefurozime Axetil, Clarithromycin, and Rifampin along with a prescription for Fluconazole thrown in the mix. In addition to those prescriptions, I had over 20 different drops, herbs and vitamins that I had to take each day. It was confusing, time consuming and very frustrating. I hate taking medicine and don't even like taking an aspirin. So for me this was pure hell at its finest. The doctor will have a list of co-infections that show up in your blood from the lab, which will help to determine what medication(s) to start with.

Many patients are low in vitamins B, D, and Omega3 fatty acids, so a daily regime of vitamins and even some herbs must be taken along with any and all prescriptions. The key here is to build up your immune system. If that is weak, your body cannot fight off the bacteria. Now Lyme disease will attack the weakest parts of your body, so for example; when I was a teenager, I went on an afterschool ski trip with many other students. That night, I took a tumble and sprained my right thumb really bad. The moment I contracted Lyme disease it found its way to the right thumb muscle tissue and has been causing severe pain and arthritic problems since. I also hurt my left knee in track and field during high school. Now, I have to be careful because the Lyme will flare up in the knee joint and it too can be unbelievably painful. So be prepared for aches and pains in areas where you had sports injuries or even prior surgeries or scar tissue.

When you start your initial treatment, you'll know within a few weeks if the medicine is doing anything. You may actually feel worse than you did before taking the meds. This is due to the bacterium getting its first dose of what I like to call "The Whoop Ass Affect". Yep, for the first time those nasty looking little cork screw bacterium that have been wreaking havoc in your body are finally getting their due. So once the medicine begins to hit them while they are cell hoping, (like twenty-one year olds bar hoping on their 21st birthday) they slowly start to die off. If however your body experiences a massive die off of the bacterium at once, you can be bed ridden and even hospitalized while going through it.

Now this may take just a few weeks to feel or it could take many months, depending on your situation. If you have a mass die off of the bacterium at once, it can make you very ill and this is unfortunately when death can occur. It takes time for the body to rid itself of the dead bacterium. Your body is basically clearing them from your blood stream, or purging. There may be medicine that your doctor prescribes that won't work well for you, and you'll know this because your doctor will tell you what symptoms may occur within days if you start having a negative reaction to it. So once again, keep that log and a pen close by at all times.

Detoxing your body will be the key to getting yourself back to good health. So you may also get Kidney and Liver detoxification drops to take a few times each day. It is necessary that you follow the doctor' guidelines on the medicines, vitamins, herbs and any other drops etc. that you are given. Yeah, you may have days where you forget to take a pill, or can't remember if you took it. I had many days where I couldn't remember I had taken the medicine just five minutes earlier, and I ended up taking it twice.

Oh well, no one is perfect especially when you have those wonderful days of "brain fog" that is so common with Lyme disease. You'll some days think you've totally lost your mind, but that's okay too. Just do the absolute best you can, but do not ever just blow off taking the medicine because you're feeling too tired to get up and take it, or because you're just tired of taking so much medicine. And yes, you will have those days.

When you first start the medicine, you may just not have the energy to do anything. I know, been there done that. But...make sure if nothing else, you at lease take a small walk each day, even if it's just to your mailbox, you need to keep moving. If you don't, the Lyme will win the battle. Lyme disease hates a well oxygenated body and cannot thrive, so the only way to keep it down is by getting oxygen in your system through some form of exercise.

If you are dealing with this very issue now, I know you'd probably like to throw something heavy at me and knock me out for sounding so flip about it. But, once again, been there done that! I was so exhausted by the time I was diagnosed that I literally could not walk up 2 steps without having to sit down and rest for several minutes, before attempting two more. This was especially enjoyable for me since I was living in a 2-story home, and the bedroom was on the second floor. So no matter how bad it is, it will keep getting worse until you mentally and physically start fighting back. I had my days where it literally took me a half hour to go up 13 steps! Be the little engine that could.

You are going to face many obstacles during your months of treatment so the best advice I can give anyone is to keep a positive attitude. I was just exhausted every day, and even while I was going through the treatment, I kept working for the first couple of months. I would go to bed exhausted. Some days I would sleep for 12 hours and wake up feeling like I hadn't slept a wink. This is normal as fatigue is a major symptom, and sleep does not make the fatigue go away. My case was pretty bad, and I had to quit my job finally to give my body time to heal. That was the most difficult thing for me.

Talk to your doctor and ask if there is anything he/she could recommend you do to get through the storm. Lyme disease will always feel like it's getting worse before you start feeling better. Once the medicine gets into your system, it's going to piss off the Lyme bacterium…and holy hell if you won't feel like a war is going on inside you! So strap your seatbelt on cause this will be a bumpy ride!

There are several things that you can do to help yourself through this shit storm. If your doctor doesn't tell you, taking *hot* Epsom Salt baths will help relieve pain and discomfort. But, you must sit in a tub of hot water, as hot as you can stand it without burning your skin. Do that every night if you need to, and try to sit in it for half hour to 45 minutes at a time. Believe me, Epsom salt could be your new best friend. In addition to the baths, you need to change your eating habits. This will be the toughest part for almost everyone. Why? Because we are all used to eating on the run, and many times we just don't get the nutrients we need from our food.

First things first, go through your cabinets and be sure the garbage can is next to you while you do. It's time to purge the snacks and all the other crap that Lyme disease loves you to eat. At this point I can hear all of you saying "are you kidding me"? Or my favorite, "I thought you were just kidding when you said this would be a total life change". No, I really meant that.

There are many *life* changes that you will have to make, and the most important is your diet. That's right, your diet. So fill that garbage can with all of the following items: (1) carbohydrates. Throw out all the processed cereal, pasta, bread, and anything that is a carbohydrate. I know you're asking yourself, "If I throw out everything that's a carbohydrate, what am I supposed to eat? I'm not done, and we're just getting started.

After you have thrown away all the carbohydrates, throw out the Sugar, coffee, tea and soda too. Oh now that's not all. Remember, keeping a positive outlook will help you heal quicker. So let us recap. You can't have carbohydrates, sugar, coffee, Tea or soda. And let us not forget to pour out the alcohol too. OMG…NOT THE ALCOHOL! I know, been there done that and it *sucks badly!*

Giving up that cold beer or glass of wine with dinner is always the hardest thing to do, especially if

---

you've been doing that for many years. So you're probably wondering why these specific items, but there are many more you cannot have.

To put it in a nutshell, you don't want to put the following items in your body because they are the foods that fuel Lyme disease. You can no longer have:

- Alcohol
- Caffeine
- Carbohydrates
- Sugar

This means no more cakes, doughnuts or deserts, and no wine or beer. I'm sure by now your mouth has dropped open and you're in disbelief. Don't worry, I had that blank look on my face too when my doctor told me this. I felt like my life was over. What the hell! I like a cold beer after a long hard day of work. I love my bread and who can't resist sugar? Carbohydrates… Everything nowadays is a carbohydrate!

So now that the initial shock wave has slapped you upside the head, lets' figure out what you can eat. All fresh fruits and veggies are good for you, especially vegetables like Spinach and Kale. I eat greens every day of my life now and I never used to. Broccoli, Swiss chard, dandelion greens, and beet greens are really good for you and the Lyme. Any green is fine. You can eat meat, and fish, chicken, pork, turkey, etc. There is no restriction on that unless you personally don't like it or can't have it because of religious beliefs. Dairy is also fine. It's really just consuming a protein diet, if any of you have ever tried that. I have learned to eat more vegetables, salads and loads of fruit. And, at the end of the day, I feel really good, and it's better for my body and mind.

Now I know it will be hard to give up everything at once, but try to get off all those Lyme loving foods within 30 days. It will help you heal quicker, and with the medicine, it will be like giving the Lyme disease a one-two punch. Exactly what needs to happen. So, learn to eat eggs or fresh fruit in the morning instead of cereal. Say good bye to Captain Crunch and Special K. It's time to dig in your heels and roll up your sleeves. Don't like eggs? Find foods that you like and eat those for breakfast, even if it's a dinner food. Just eat healthy.

This is real life hitting home right now. This isn't Kansas and no Dorothy, you cannot click you heels 3x and wake up cured. This is your new life. And not for nothing, but it's a better life. It's the way every person should be eating every day. It's a healthier, more nutritious way. And what's so bad about having a good salmon salad or chicken salad for lunch or dinner? Why not eat what's good for you? I've been eating like a queen, and I'm enjoying it!

I am trying new recipes all the time, and I cook with olive oil which is extremely healthy as well. You have to make the change if you want to live a normal life. I've been off medication for several months now, and still, if I eat a bag of potato chips or have a soda, I'm like a pile of crap the next day. A glass of wine will put me on the sofa for 3 days. It does affect me and it feeds the Lyme every time I allow myself to go off course. It makes me lethargic and I feel very fatigued if I don't eat properly. I have several different smoothie recipes that I make which are wonderful. I make them for breakfast or whenever I feel like it. You will see those later in the book. Even if you're not a good cook, everyone can make a salad or throw some fruit or vegetables into a blender. And, once you get it through your thick head that this is your new lifestyle, you will become more interested in learning what to make for yourself. It's time to expand your horizons.

Now, you've changed your eating habits (or are in the process) and you are getting exercise every day, what else is there? Stress control and meditation. Stress is a huge factor in Lyme. If you have a stressful job, it will reflect on your health, that's just a given fact. So can you imagine how much worse off your body will be if you allow the stress around you to creep into your soul? You are trying to recover from Lyme disease, not have a relapse! Yes, stress can cause you to relapse, just like your diet and exercise programs can too.

Must I remind you again that Lyme disease is a "game changer"? It is a life change for all of us who want to live. So be consistent in all phases of these changes. If you fall of the wagon and eat crappy snack foods after a week of eating healthy, your body will feel it immediately. Mediation can help you to stay focused and remain calm which is important. By spending just ten minutes a day in complete quiet where you just let you brain relax, the results are amazing. Now it doesn't count if you spend that ten minutes going over the daily work load or a conversation you had in your mind. Let your mind be idol for those ten minutes. You deserve that time, so take it. If you can take more than ten minutes…do, but get in at least ten precious minutes of meditation each day.

This might sound like a cliché, but it is important that your mind, body and spirit be working as one. If just one area is out of whack, it throws the entire system off. So to get healthy and remain healthy you must be consistent in all areas. Eat right, exercise, meditate and keep stress out of your life.

Once you get the ball rolling you'll find out that making these changes really isn't so hard. And after a month or two, it will become second nature and you won't even remember the old way of living. But most importantly, you will feel the immense difference in your entire body. A good difference for sure.

I will promise you two things; one, if you follow these guide rules you will feel great and live a fairly normal life style. Even if you can't do everything you did before you got Lyme disease. Second, if you don't follow these guide rules you will have a very long drawn out recovery and possibly no recovery at all. These life changes must happen if you want to live and stay on this planet a bit longer. Believe me if you don't, your life span will be cut short by many years. People are dying from Lyme disease, and this is no joke. If you want to live, suck it up and make the changes or start planning your funeral early.

Now I don't want to scare people, but sometimes you have to put the match in front of their face before they can see the fire. Don't be lazy or complacent, it's your life…enjoy every moment you have here. And take time to literally smell the roses. Use this as an eye opener to what is going on out there that you have been missing for so long.

My life isn't perfect, but then what fun would it be if it were? I can't do many of the same things I did prior to my Lyme diagnosis, but overall, I'm living a pretty good life and I enjoy the changes that I had to make. It actually made me appreciate the little things so much more. And since I don't like to sugarcoat anything, I'll tell you that at the age now of 51, I am starting over. Yes, I am completely starting my life over from square one. Lyme disease wiped me out financially and it brought 20 pounds of extra weight to my ass that I really am having a hard time getting rid of. Yes, you will gain weight with Lyme disease. Once you get on the medication and you begin to heal, start to exercise but give your body time to adjust and the weight will come off, but it will be a slow process.

What most people don't know is this; most medical professionals believe that Lyme disease can be cured with just 2-4 weeks' worth of antibiotics. NOT!!! And because of that crap way of thinking, the insurance companies will only pay for that much treatment. The rest is ala you and out of your pocket. So don't expect your insurance company to ante up big on those doctor bills because that's nothing but a pipe dream. Many insurance companies don't even believe Lyme disease exists! The truth is, they don't want to believe it or they'll have to pay more out for treatment. So prepare yourself for out of pocket expenditures of medicine and even doctor visits.

There were many months where I was spending over $2,000. 00 between refills of the medicines, (some over $200 each) my doctor visits, and the blood tests. Oh yeah, be prepared to take lots of blood tests too. This is the only way the doctor can determine if they are curing the co-infections. I took blood work every 4-6 weeks. My first set of blood tests cost me $1169.00 out of pocket. That was with a 66% discount because I didn't have insurance.

And yes, I almost shit myself when the receptionist told me the price. She said it so matter of fact, like it was no big deal. I had to play it off cool so I wrote the check and went running to the bank to transfer every penny I had into the checking so the check wouldn't bounce. After all, the blood was already drawn so I couldn't back out now. If you have insurance, it will cover only a hand full of these tests before you reach your limit. And, if you have co-pay, it will start to add up fast.

For those of you who don't have health insurance...don't panic and think that you have no options. The affordable health care act will now help those who need this treatment. It was tough having to come up with the money every time I needed a new prescription or had to go see the doctor who charged $575.00 per hour of visit. But, if you get the diagnosis from your first visit, you can holistically get it under control, but the treatment time is at least double of that with prescriptions. Either way, a change in diet and exercise will help you through the process.

Looking back, I literally spent every penny I made on my Lyme disease, but it was worth it, and I was fortunate to have been able to bring in money during my recovery. I worked the first two months and then had to quit my job. I couldn't collect disability because the company I worked for fought it and won. Even though I got the infection while working, it was impossible to prove that. This left me holding the bag. I was in construction and wore my tool belt every day, swinging hammers for a living and teaching others how to build homes. After the first two months of treatment, I could no longer swing the hammer.

I knew it was time to quit when the hammer flew out of my hand and almost hit my co-worker in the head. I literally could not grip the hammer anymore because the Lyme had crept into the muscle of my right hand and left me somewhat useless. I can pick up a hammer today, but I can't do what I did just 3 years ago. And that's ok, because I'm still here and can do other things. Lyme disease is a *life change,* but it gave me, the opportunity to reinvent myself again so I can pursue other ventures. That's how you need to look at any disease. Don't let it take your life or your spirit away, just fight it and do something else. You might wonder why you didn't try it sooner.

Since being taken off the medicine, I have moved from the east coast back to the Midwest. This was a good move for my recovery. The east coast was nothing but a stressful hustle and bustle every day. The stress was keeping me from recovering as quickly as I needed and wanted to, and after 29 years out east, I hung up my Jersey roots and came back to a more relaxed way of life. Now certainly not everyone will need to move to recover from Lyme, but for me, it was the right decision.

For those of you, who don't have thousands of dollars to spend on recovery, just know that you can do a lot just by eating healthy and getting enough exercise. Remember, Lyme is a lifelong disease. Yes getting on antibiotics will make a huge difference, but I could have said no to the prescriptions and concentrated on vitamins, herbs and life style change to get myself feeling better. Not all people believe in taking medicine. You can get better by changing what you do and what you eat. Talk to a specialist to find out what treatment is right for you based on your circumstances. But no matter what you decide, you must change your lifestyle. Once you do, you will begin the healing process and be able to continue living and loving life.

Now again, Lyme will be in your body forever. But, to live with it and keep it in a dormant state, you have to starve it. By this I mean; don't eat the foods that it thrives on. Refer to the list of items listed earlier in the book. Don't get lazy and stop exercising or you will see the dormant bacterium rear its ugly head and start wreaking havoc again. Your body cannot handle going back and forth. Eat right, cheat, eat right, cheat, exercise don't exercise. You need to be consistent with everything you do. Get a routine going that works for you, and just repeat it day after day. This is absolutely imperative to keeping the Lyme in a dormant (sleeping) stage.

Chapter Eight:
The correlation between Lyme disease and infant Autism

Over the last 10-15 years, infant autism has been on a steady rise. This had researchers puzzled until just recently. The LIA (Lyme Induced Autism) foundation was established in 2006 by a group of parents who suspected the connection but also realized the need for research on the matter. The foundation is led by one of those parents named Tami Duncan, a mother of an autistic child.

Doctors Charles Ray Jones M.D. and Warren Levin, M.D. both gave talks about their research finding at a conference held April 12, 2008 in Fort Lee, New Jersey. Doctor Jones had treated over 10,000 children with Lyme disease and told his audience that a good many of the children he had treated, were found to have had autism-spectrum disorder. Doctor Levin spoke about an autistic child he treated, who tested positive for Lyme disease. After that, Doctor Levin began checking all of the autistic patients and nine in a row tested positive for the disease.

Now many of you may be saying well, that's not enough scientific evidence to prove the two are related. It is true that much more research still needs to be done, but being a Lyme disease patient myself, I will say that's pretty staggering news. And even since the 2008 conference, the number of autistic children who have tested positive for Lyme has increased tremendously. Remember, Lyme disease is the "great imitator". I agree with many doctors who believe the Lyme bacterium is being passed along to the fetus before birth, and this is the outcome.

This is why it's all too important for any woman who is pregnant or contemplating pregnancy to get blood work taken before having a baby. There are too many women who don't even realize they have Lyme disease, and therefore passing on a death sentence to their unborn child when it could have been prevented. I think women owe it to the unborn to have these simple tests taken so you can confront the issue head on. Better to be safe than sorry.

I'm going to refer back to my girlfriend Linda. Well before being diagnosed with Lyme, Linda got married and became pregnant with her first child. A few years later she gave birth to twins. She is very concerned about the health of her 3 boys and rightfully so, especially since one of them is showing all the signs of Lyme. He has the fatigue, brain fog, sleepless nights especially when he eats any junk food before bedtime. Linda has kept strict logs of what her family eats. They are a very healthy family and eat next to no junk food, which is very surprising with 3 boys.

On occasion however, the boys will ask for potato chips or other snacks so she will oblige, since it only happens once a month. Hey, kids got to be kids you know? You must change your diet with Lyme disease, however, if you get a craving for something every now and then...go ahead and live a little! But, be warned that you may feel like someone stomped on you the next day or for several days after. So each time her boys have any junk food, she notices changes in their moods, mannerisms and especially their energy level.

Her one son cannot sleep or function well in school the next day after eating those potato chips. Each time he goes through the fatigue and brain fog,

Linda has to remind him that he just can't eat the junk food.

At present, the doctor is aware that he has Lyme, but because he is still young, they want to treat it holistically before trying prescriptions. Linda says as long as he eats fruits, vegetables and a higher protein diet, he seems fine. All her boys are very active in school and sports, and any young kid who has to miss games or sports because he can't get out of bed just becomes unhappy. So her son has decided that he would rather feel good and play sports with his buddies than be in bed feeling lethargic. It's all about diet and exercise, and when he has both in check, he seems perfectly normal.

She has also seen some signs of Lyme in her other two boys, but not as severe as the first. So keep in mind again that each case is different. What affects one person may not affect another, or at least in the same manner. If you're not sure if an ache or pain is part of Lyme disease, do some research or ask a specialist. There are so many different symptoms that it is impossible to list all of them. As for infant autism, it's hard to believe that so many innocent children are being affected by this government designed and produced disease. Those kids didn't do anything wrong, but their lives will be permanently affected by it. This is what angers me the most.

Why shouldn't our government be held responsible for this epidemic? And who knows if those scientists realized that even their own flesh and blood could be infected by Lyme or infant autism. Life can be tough enough without having diseases thrown at us, using us as guinea pigs for their science projects. Because Lyme disease is such an epidemic globally, I feel that blood testing for Lyme and its co-infections should be done on every person automatically. It should be part of every physical or check up. This would help to get proper numbers of those infected so scientists have a clear idea of the severity with this disease.

If we know what we're dealing with in real time numbers, it's easier to treat and get under control. The longer this goes on, the worse it will be, making it unstoppable. So be sure to do your part and get tested for Lyme and its co-infections so you and your family can stay safe and healthy.

Chapter Nine
How to remove ticks safely from your body.

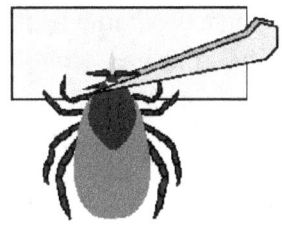

(Photo: LDF)

The proper way to remove a tick from your body is shown to the left. Use a tweezers. Be sure you place the tweezers as close to the mouth as possible. Gently pull back so the tick releases itself. Do not tug or the body will break off and leave the head below the skin. Remove the entire tick at one time.

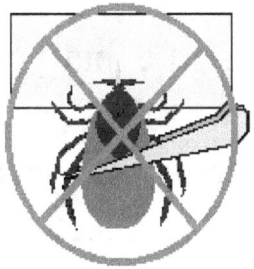

(Photo: LDF)

Never grab a tick by the body. Once the body is engorged with blood, if you squeeze it, the infected blood will go into the blood stream. This is what you want to avoid at all costs.

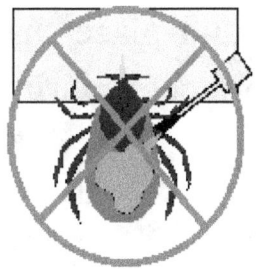

(Photo: LDF)

Never put rubbing alcohol, nail polish, or petroleum jelly, on the tick to try to smother it or back it out of the skin. This too will make it release the infected blood into your blood stream.

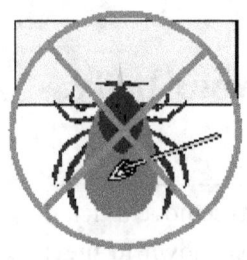

(Photo: LDF)

Never use a lit match on a tick. Trying to burn a tick off the body will allow the infected blood back into your blood stream. Never twist, turn or try to jerk the tick from the skin. Gently and slowly remove it so the entire tick comes out in one piece. Then, rinse the area with soap and water to disinfect the bite as best as you can. If possible, take the tick with you in a jar to your doctor. See a doctor immediately after the bite.

If you are not sure what a tick looks like, but you suspect you have one, you can send it to the Insect Diagnostic Laboratory at Cornell University. The cost is $25 per specimen, and they do not test for infections within the tick. They only verify that it is or is not a tick. Never send the tick in alcohol, as it is illegal to do so. Place the tick in an envelope and place that envelope inside a bubble envelope to protect it during shipping.

Your local county health office should also be able to assist you as to where you can send the tick sample, perhaps closer to your home. Be sure to ask for pricing before you send it, as labs will vary in price.

Be sure to send it along with a note asking them to verify it is a tick, and make certain you leave a phone number or address where they can contact you with their results.

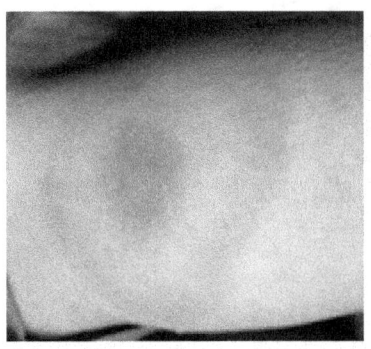

(Photo: LDF) Bull's eye rash

Although many people never see the bull's eye on their skin, the photo to the left shows a perfect example of a bull's eye. There will be a red circle in the center where the bite actually occurred, with a larger red ring around it. If you do see the bull's eye, get to a doctor immediately for evaluation.

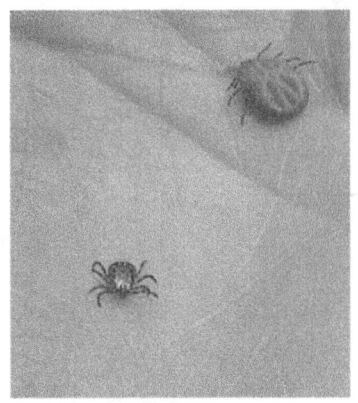

(Photo: LDF) Dog ticks

The photo to the left shows 2 ticks. The bottom tick is flat which means it has not yet filled with blood. If they are removed before the body becomes engorged, it's a good possibility that you have not been infected. The upper tick is engorged, which means it has been feeding for perhaps a few days. By this point the infected blood has been passed into the blood stream.

Page 91

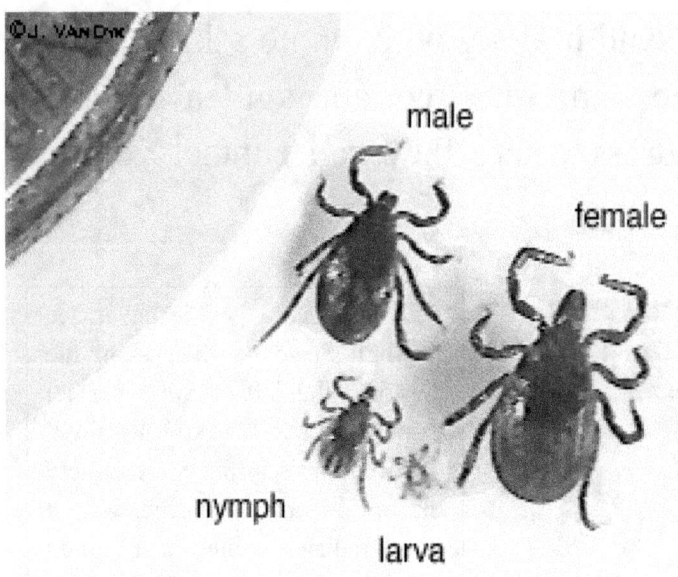

(Photo: LDF) Stages of a tick

The photo to the left shows the different stages of a tick's life. Bottom right is the larva; to the left is the nymph, then male and female. Nymph and female stages are the infectious stages for tick bites.

Chapter Ten:
How to live with Chronic Lyme disease

Chronic Lyme disease will be a big part of your life once you are through the initial treatment. It will be like having arthritis, but the aches and pains could be more severe. It's important to keep it under control so it doesn't run your life.

You already know that you have to change your diet and get plenty of exercise. Your body needs rest as well, so getting a solid eight hours of sleep every night will help you maintain the basics. In addition to the life changes that you already have to make, you will need to think about *post Lyme treatment*. What I mean by post Lyme treatment, is the secondary care that you will need once you are off your prescriptions.

Don't get cocky and think that you're fine just because the doctor tells you it's time to stop taking all those pills. Yes, it's great that you finally won't have that headache to deal with every day, and you'll save loads of money that you had to spend each month on the medicine. But, now you have to focus on long term care. You should see an optimologist and have your eyes checked. Why? Because Lyme will attack the eyes, and if you notice your eye sight suddenly going down the toilet, make sure you get it checked. Be sure you call around and find an eye doctor who has experience with Lyme disease. They're out there you just have to find them.

There is medicine to help with the vision problems, and it's quite possible you will need eye drops or something else to keep it from getting worse. Don't delay. I know a woman who almost went blind and had she not gotten her eyes checked when she did, she would have lost sight completely. The doctor put her on two different types of eye drops and low and behold, her vision is doing just fine now.

In addition to eye health, lets' talk a little bit about possible acupuncture. It really does work, and after just a few treatments, the aches and pains subside. Lyme does a number on the shoulders and lower back. Many people get Chronic Lyme Arthritis in the joints such as the knees, elbows and even the hips. I still have those pains and when Epsom Salt baths just don't do the trick, you'll thank me for telling you this.

One of my biggest pains is my right thumb tissue. If you recall me saying earlier, I sprained it terribly on an after school ski trip when I was a teenager. I've never really had problems with it until I got Lyme disease. Now, I have pain quite often. It gets very swollen when we have changes in the weather. Acupuncture is the key for long term care and good health.

If you look around, you'll probably find an acupuncturist who has treated Lyme patients, but it's not necessary. A good acupuncturist will be able to help you either way. The first time I went, I was blown away by the difference it made in my body. The doctor I went to was recommended by my mother-in-law. Believe it or not, the man was legally blind! Yeah, I couldn't believe it myself, but he held my wrist and like a psychic he told me about ailments I had experienced without any knowledge or information from me. He was amazing!

The cool thing is, I've always believed in alternative and holistic medicines. I don't like taking pills. Doctors nowadays seem to like pushing pills for everything, and people are just over medicated. I know a few doctors personally, and they made it very clear that they get large monthly bonuses from the pharmaceutical companies for pushing their products. They tell me they need to supplement their incomes because insurances are sky high.

Going to an acupuncturist won't be a regular event. Most times, you will go for 2-4 visits and then not go back again until your aches or pains return, if they do. For me, three treatments did the job on my lower back. Some people go once a month just for maintenance. It's a really good idea, but let the doctor tell you what he/she believes your treatment should be. You could look at it like you do a dentist. Most people get their teeth cleaned every 6 months for good oral hygiene and have yearly check-ups for everything else. That's what an acupuncturist can do for you as well, maintain good long term health.

Lots of people go to Chiropractors and message therapists to manage pain and that too is fine. Maintain your body like you would a Jaguar or a Rolls Royce automobile. You don't want to forget about changing the oil, or it could cause serious engine problems down the road, and cost tons of money. But if you keep it running in tip top shape, the car will last many, many years without replacing any major parts. We don't want to worry about replacing parts! So, keep your body in tip top shape, and you can and will put the Lyme to rest for a very long time.

Okay, I know I'm giving you loads of things to remember, so lets' recap to have a clear understanding. Are you ready?

First, change your diet. Get rid of Carbohydrates, caffeine, sugar and alcohol. Eat fresh and organic whenever possible. Start an exercise program (one that you can do each day that you won't dread). Get at least 8 hours of sleep each night. See an eye doctor to make certain your eyesight has not been affected by Lyme disease.

Make an appointment with an acupuncturist to maintain the chronic arthritic aches and pains. If you also see a chiropractor or message therapist, continue as they can also do wonders for your body. And finally, keep an upbeat attitude. If you think negative and surround yourself with negativity, you will find that more and more of what you don't want (negativity) will show up. Be careful what you wish for. Put out good mojo and you will receive good mojo.

Chapter Eleven:
Food you will love and Lyme disease will hate.

I like eggs and bacon and toast. But, I'm not supposed to have bread, because it's a carbohydrate. So what else can I eat for breakfast now that I can't have bread or cereal? If you like eggs, bacon, sausage then eat it. I don't want it every day either, so I will switch up the morning meal routine with yogurt and/or fruit. Many mornings I'll eat a small bowl of cottage cheese with pineapple in it, or fresh fruit.

If you can't have dairy and don't eat bacon and eggs, how about trying a morning smoothie? They are so good for you and are packed with loads of vitamins and nutrients. There are even mornings where I make myself a small piece of Salmon. I love Salmon. How about Lox without the bagel? You need to be creative and try some new things. I never used to make smoothies until my girlfriend gave me a taste of hers one day. I was hooked! I have several breakfast recipes for smoothies and drink concoctions that I make quite a bit. They are delicious and very refreshing.

Lunches are pretty easy. Salads are great and very nutritious. Having a piece of grilled chicken, salmon or beef over the salad makes a great meal. You can put a wonderful salad together at home to take with you for lunch in just a few minutes of your time. If you're not a salad eater, but love your sub sandwiches, you can still have all the goodies that come on the sub, just do without the bread. I did this when I was on the Atkins diet and it was great. After a week, I didn't miss the bread. Even a plate of roasted veggies makes a great lunch, or fresh veggies and dip. Eat healthy but do it with things that you like. Not everyone likes eating celery with dip…o.k., so how about asparagus, beets, carrots, tomatoes, radishes, onions, zucchini, broccoli? There are a million great vegetables that you can eat roasted or fresh. Get a juicer and make a great nutritious drink that's packed with vitamins and will fill you up at lunch.

For those of you who are seafood eaters, preparing a piece of fish to take with you to work or to eat at home is very quick and simple. I love tuna out of a can, and the same with sardines or any type of fish. My ancestors were Scandinavian so that's where the fish thing comes from for me. Soups are great all year round. I make great summer time soups that are excellent. Some are hot and some are cold but all are wonderful and filling. And for those people who like lighter lunches, how about slices of your favorite cheese with a crisp apple? Try peanut butter and honey layered over a sliced banana…it is so good!

Lots of people will eat yogurt or cottage cheese with pineapple in it for lunch. It just depends on your likes and dislikes, but you can still enjoy most of the things you once ate, they'll just be prepared and presented a bit differently than you are used to.

How about dinner? For those of you who love meat and potatoes like me, you can still have the meat, but go light on the potatoes as they are a starch (carbohydrate). How about cooked cauliflower mashed like potatoes? I tried it once, it's called cauliflower mash, and it is really good. Fish, chicken, beef, turkey, lamb, or any meat is fine. Be careful not to use bread crumbs or if you do, very minimal for some of your dishes. Now, if you are a big pasta eater you're going to have a few issues. You can have all the clams, seafood, meat etc. and even load up on the gravy, just stay away from the pasta! I never said it was going to be easy to make all the changes to your diet, but after a few weeks you'll become comfortable with your new meals, and it will be easier. I also know that you will have much more energy when you change your diet. When you begin to starve the Lyme disease, you will feel your body fighting from within. But hang in there and don't give up.

It will seem like the Lyme will be screaming "FEED ME"! You will find yourself hungry more often because your diet will be mostly protein and your body will burn it off more rapidly than if you were eating carbohydrates. But, again, you'll have loads of energy, and you'll find yourself sleeping sound and through the entire night. You will have to try new things, for example; I never ate Kale in my life until my doctor recommended it. Once I tried it, I was hooked. I eat Kale at least once a day and sometimes twice. Be open and use this as your reason to expand your food horizon.

So below are some recipes that I learned to make from my own research. Some were given to me by friends and my doctor.

Breakfast:

I love to make nutritious but tasty drinks in the morning. One of my favorites is the Pear/Ginger drink. I use a juicer but if you don't have one, put everything in a blender or food processor.

Pear/Ginger Juice

1 fresh pear halved and seeds removed. Or ½ cup of your favorite juice.
1 large cucumber cut into quarters, length wise.
4-6 stalks of celery. Cut off the bottoms and leaves from the top.
(1) 1" piece of ginger root peeled.

Juice it all together and drink! Or, throw it into the blender or processor, but peel the pear and cucumber before mixing. Add ¼ cup of water only to the blender or food processor. If the drink is too thick, add water until it is at the right consistency for you. This drink is so refreshing. You can substitute a real pear for pear juice or any other fruit juice.

I also use this same recipe but if I don't have a pear, I'll use a mango, or guava juice and even watermelon juice and it's wonderful.

Green Drink

1 cup of fresh spinach, lettuce, kale, Swiss chard, beet greens, or a mix of several together.
4 stalks of celery
1 large cucumber quartered
½ cup of coconut water

Juice all and drink, or place in a blender or food processor and liquefy. If it is too thick, add water slowly until you have the consistency that is right for you.

Veggie drink

½ cup of water
2 carrots quartered lengthwise
1 cucumber quartered lengthwise
2 stalks of celery
½ cup of spinach
½ cup of orange juice or apple juice.
Mix and serve cold.

Yogurt Smoothie

½ cup of vanilla yogurt

½ cup of berries (blueberries, raspberries, black berries or a mix. Any berries will be fine).

½ cup of coconut milk

Mix in a blender and enjoy cold.

Tropical Smoothie

½ cup of your banana flavored yogurt

½ cup of Ice

½ cup of coconut milk

½ cup of tropical fruit; mango, papaya, guava, kiwi

Blend all together well in a blender and drink cold. Delicious!

Lunch:

Strawberry almond salad with red wine vinaigrette

Take 1 cup of your favorite lettuce or make a mix of several types.

Slice up 6 large strawberries and place on top of the greens.

Add a small hand full of sliced almonds.

Add ¼ cup of blue cheese

Top with raspberry vinaigrette

Pear/Walnut Salad

1 cup of salad greens
1 pear peeled and sliced and placed on top of the lettuce
1 small hand full of walnuts tossed on top
3 small slices of goat cheese tossed on top
Sprinkle with balsamic vinaigrette and enjoy

Super Food Salad

Mix equal parts of spinach, beet greens, kale, Swiss chard and collard greens. Top with your favorite toppings and salad dressing. The inside of your body will scream in delight for so many good vitamins and nutrients in one meal!

There are millions of salads you can make so experiment and have fun.

Quick Salmon Lunch

1 piece of Salmon
1 tbsp. olive oil + additional for the bottom of your pan
1 tsp lite soy sauce
1 shallot sliced white and green portions

Mix the olive oil and soy sauce together and stir until mixed. Oil the bottom of your pan and place the salmon skin side down. Pour the olive oil/soy sauce mix over the top of the salmon. Toss the shallots along the sides of the pan and let cook with the Salmon for two minutes. Flip salmon over and cook another two minutes. Stir the shallots. After 2 minutes, place the salmon on a plate, skin side down and spoon shallots over the top and serve with your favorite vegetable.

Cooked Kale

In a skillet, add 2 tbsp. of water and a bunch of washed kale leaves (stems removed). Steam for just 2 minutes covered until the leaves are wilted and the water has evaporated from the pan. Place the kale in a large bowl, add shredded parmesan cheese and sprinkle about 2 tbsp. of olive oil over the top. Serve immediately.

Kale can be eaten as a meal or served as a side with your entre. You will love Kale, and maybe find that you'll make it as your main breakfast meal some days. I got to the point where I was eating Kale at least once a day, and if I didn't, my body would crave it. The vitamin K is so good for your body.

Kale Chips (Snack)

1 bunch of Kale washed, dried, and stems removed. (Use leaves only)
Olive oil for tossing
Adobo seasoning.

Place kale leaves in a large bowl and coat with olive oil. Lay them on a pan side by side. Sprinkle Adobo seasoning lightly on top of each leaf and bake for 10-15 minutes at 350 degrees until kale becomes crispy and even slightly burnt. Cool and enjoy like potato chips!

Have a sub sandwich without the bread…it's basically a salad on a bun when you really look at it. So without the bread, you place everything on a plate and it becomes a salad.

Cottage cheese and fruit are also good for lunch if you like lighter meals.

Yogurt smoothies are not just for breakfast. They are refreshing at lunch time too. If you are a fast food junkie, go and get your burger or hotdog. Just throw away the bun! You will not only feel so much better and have more energy, but you'll find yourself losing weight,

Get some healthy snacks for yourself, like nuts, raisins, and dried fruits. Make your own ice pops with fresh fruit juice and eat those instead of ice cream, candy or chips.

Try not to eat too late, as your body cannot digest the food once you lie down. This will disturb your sleep pattern and can cause stress on your body.

Try eating lighter dinners as well. Seafood is always light and easy to digest. So try having a nice piece of fish with a simple vegetable for dinner. I love tea after my meal but caffeine is out of the question. So, to get the best of both worlds, I grow and dry my own peppermint and I steep that in hot water and the green colored caffeine free tea is wonderful.

Grilled chicken is also a light meal if you pair it with a simple vegetable. You don't have to be an amazing cook to eat well. If you just do some simple planning you can make some great recipes in just a few short minutes.

It's important to keep your body cleansing from the inside out. In lots of third world countries, people eat loads of hot peppers and hot sauce which kills off bacteria in the body. Lyme cannot flourish in an atmosphere that is filled with good properties. So what is considered good properties? Well, oxygen is the main property that Lyme disease cannot live with. *Any disease* will thrive in a body that is lacking nutrients, vitamins and minerals. When a body is lacking these properties, that means the oxygen level is low and any disease will grow and flourish. Add back in all the good stuff that the body is missing and needs, and the disease starts to die off because it can't feed in a good environment.

My girlfriend gave me this recipe to help detox the body and to ward off bacteria. Try it and if you follow this protocol every day for a week, you'll find that if you stop taking it, your body will crave more.

Jalapeno pepper paste

3/4 lb of jalapeno peppers (Remove the stems and toss in a blender whole).
Add ½ cup olive oil.

When it is all ground up, add the following:

1 bunch of cilantro and blend
1 bunch of parsley and blend
1 Tbsp Tahini and blend

Add 1 can of chick peas (drained) 18oz.

Mix all together and refrigerate. This will last at least 2 weeks. Eat 3 tbsp. 2-3 times a day with rice chips or veggies. This will keep your body from building up toxins and bacteria. It is an excellent cleansing agent.

So let's look again at the bad: Low oxygen, yeast, carbohydrates, caffeine, alcohol, sugar, low levels of vitamins B, D and Omega fatty3 acids, no exercise and stress. Sounds like a bomb waiting to go off!

Now lets' look at the good: High levels of oxygen, exercise, loads of vitamins and minerals, healthy meals, good sound sleep, low or no stress levels, acupuncture, message every now and then. Sound like a party going on here!

Keep these in mind as you go through your battle with Lyme disease. And use these same principals for any ailments in your life. Eat, live and stay healthy through diet and exercise and your body (your Rolls Royce) will run for many, many years to come.

Informational Sites

ILADS (International Lyme and Associated Diseases Society)
www.ILADS.org

CDC (Centers for Disease Control)
www.cdc.gov

ALDF (American Lyme Disease Foundation)
www.aldf.com

Through my own research, I have found the ILADS organization to be the best site for me. You can find Lyme specialists in your area, and many informational sources of new research and findings on this site. More and more studies are taking place every day somewhere on the planet. I believe at some point we will find a cure, I just hope we find it before too many innocent people die.

Check out the ILADS Lyme Wall. See photos of people who have Lyme disease, and read a little story about each of them. The ILADS website has the most up to date research on Lyme disease. The CDC however, although it has opinions from doctors, there are doctors who still believe that Lyme disease does not exist within the CDC family.

I hope you have found this information helpful to you in your quest for knowledge about Lyme disease. Please follow me on my website at: www.lifewithlymedisease.com for all the current information and research that is taking place around the globe. Live Love and Be Happy every day that you are on this planet.

Sincerely,
Kathryn Nedved Hoffman
Lyme disease survivor

Don't forget to read about the important people who helped make this book possible.

www.lifewithlymedisease.com

Acknowledgements:

I would like to thank all the Lyme patients who came forward and opened up their hearts to tell me their stories, and allowed me to utilize the information to help other Lyme patients through the writing of this book.

I would also like to thank LDF for the photos of ticks and bulls-eye bite that I used in the book, as well as Istock for my cover photo.

Most of all, I would like to thank my friend Linda for inspiring me with her story. It was Linda who put me in touch with the Lyme Specialist in NJ who in turn, helped me to get back on track and most importantly, showed me how to live with "Chronic Lyme Disease".

I would like to dedicate this book to all those Lyme patients suffering with this terrible disease, and to those who have given the greatest sacrifice…their life.

In fond memory of Lilly Hudson.

I know that those who read this book will get some good information out of it. As more and more information becomes available, and more research is done, I will post new findings and research results on my website at: www.lifewithlymedisease.com.

Please feel free to visit the website as often as you like. Keep informed on this epidemic and help spread the word.

www.ingramcontent.com/pod-product-compliance
Lightning Source LLC
Chambersburg PA
CBHW070928290526
45795CB00001B/471